# WRECK THIS JOURNAL

# TO CREATE IS TO DESTROY

BY KERI SMITH

PARTICULAR
BOOKS

# PARTICULAR BOOKS

PUBLISHED BY THE PENGUIN GROUP

PENGUIN BOOKS LTD, 80 STRAND, LONDON WC2R ORL, ENGLAND

PENGUIN GROUP (USA) INC, 375 HUDSON STREET, NEW YORK, NEW YORK 10014, USA

PENGUIN GROUP (CANADA), 90 EGLINTON AVENUE EAST, SUITE 700, TORONTO, ONTARIO, CANADA M4P 2Y3

(A DIVISION OF PEARSON PENGUIN CANADA INC.)

PENGUIN IRELAND, 25 ST STEPHENS GREEN, DUBLIN 2, IRELAND (A DIVISION OF PENGUIN BOOKS LTD)

PENGUIN GROUP (AUSTRALIA), 707 COLLINS STREET, MELBOURNE, VICTORIA 3008, AUSTRALIA

(A DIVISION OF PEARSON AUSTRALIA GROUP PTY LTD)

PENGUIN BOOKS INDIA PVT LTD, 11 COMMUNITY CENTRE, PANCHSHEEL PARK, NEW DELHI – 110 017, INDIA

PENGUIN GROUP (NZ), 67 APOLLO DRIVE, ROSEDALE, AUCKLAND 0632, NEW ZEALAND

(A DIVISION OF PEARSON NEW ZEALAND LTD)

PENGUIN BOOKS (SOUTH AFRICA) (PTY) LTD, BLOCK D, ROSEBANK OFFICE PARK, 181 JAN SMUTS AVENUE,

PARKTOWN NORTH, GAUTENG 2193, SOUTH AFRICA

PENGUIN BOOKS LTD, REGISTERED OFFICES: 80 STRAND, LONDON WC2R ORL, ENGLAND

www.PENGUIN.COM

FIRST PUBLISHED IN THE UNITED STATES OF AMERICA BY PENGUIN GROUP (USA) INC, 2007

FIRST PUBLISHED IN GREAT BRITAIN BY PARTICULAR BOOKS 2010

THIS EDITION PUBLISHED WITH FURTHER MATERIAL 2012

COPYRIGHT © KERI SMITH, 2007, 2012

ART AND DESIGN BY KERI SMITH

PRINTED IN ENGLAND BY CLAYS LTD, ST IVES PLC

ISBN: 978-0-141-97896-3

www.greenpenguin.co.uk

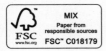

**WARNING:** DURING THE PROCESS OF THIS BOOK YOU WILL GET DIRTY. YOU MAY FIND YOURSELF COVERED IN PAINT, OR ANY OTHER NUMBER OF FOREIGN SUBSTANCES. YOU WILL GET WET. YOU MAY BE ASKED TO DO THINGS YOU QUESTION. YOU MAY GRIEVE FOR THE PERFECT STATE THAT YOU FOUND THE BOOK IN. YOU MAY BEGIN TO SEE CREATIVE DESTRUCTION EVERYWHERE. YOU MAY BEGIN TO LIVE MORE RECKLESSLY.

**Acknowledgments** This book was made with the help of the following people: my husband, Jefferson Pitcher, who provides constant inspiration for living a full and daring life (some of his ideas ended up here). Thanks to the talented artists Steve Lambert and Cynthia Yardley-Lambert who helped me brainstorm ideas during a lecture on contemporary art. To my editor at Perigee, Meg Leder, who embraced and believed in this project from the beginning, your thoughts and sensitivity left me with so much gratitude. To my agent, Faith Hamlin, for continuing to believe in my artistic/creative vision. Thanks also to Corita Kent, John Cage, Ross Mendes, Brenda Veland, Bruno Munari, and Charles and Rae Eames, whose ideas and perceptions continue to rip me wide open.

Dedicated to perfectionists all over the world.

THIS BOOK BELONGS TO:

*Serena Turtle*
_____
WRITE YOUR NAME IN WHITE.


_____
WRITE YOUR NAME ILLEGIBLY.


_____
WRITE YOUR NAME IN TINY LETTERS.

serena Turtle
_____
WRITE YOUR NAME BACKWARD.

eltrut aneres
_____
WRITE YOUR NAME VERY FAINTLY.



Serena Turtle
_____
WRITE YOUR NAME USING LARGE LETTERS.

SERENA TURTLE
_____
ADDRESS


_____
PHONE NUMBER

* NOTE: IF FOUND, FLIP TO A PAGE RANDOMLY,
         FOLLOW THE INSTRUCTIONS, THEN RETURN.

INSTRUCTIONS

1. Carry this with you everywhere you go.

2. Follow the instructions on every page.

3. Order is not important.

4. Instructions are open to interpretation.

5. Experiment.
(work against your better judgment.)

# materials

ideas
gum
glue
dirt
saliva
water
weather
garbage
plant life
pencil/pen
needle & thread
stamps
stickers
sticky things
sticks
spoons
comb
twist tie
ink
paint
grass
detergent
grease
tears
crayons

smells
hands
string
ball
unpredictability
spontaneity
photos
newspaper
white things
office supplies
wax
found items
stapler
food
tea/coffee
emotions
fears
shoes
matches
biology
scissors
tape
time
happenstance
gumption
sharp things

# ADD YOUR OWN PAGE NUMBERS.

STARTING HERE

# CRACK THE SPINE.

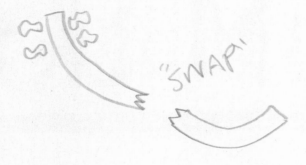

LEAVE THIS PAGE
BLANK
ON PURPOSE.

# STAND HERE.

(WIPE YOUR FEET, JUMP UP AND DOWN.)

POUR, SPILL, *drip*, SPIT, *fling* YOUR COFFEE

HERE.

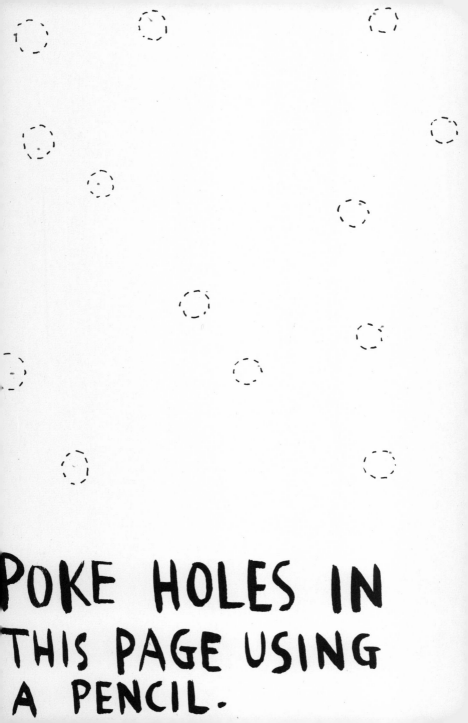

POKE HOLES IN
THIS PAGE USING
A PENCIL.

# DRAW FAT LINES AND THIN.

PUSHING REALLY HARD WITH THE PENCIL.

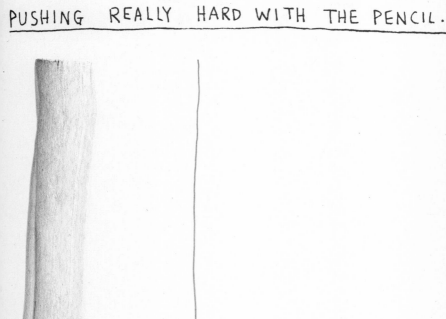

THIS PAGE IS FOR HANDPRINTS
OR FINGERPRINTS.
GET THEM DIRTY THEN PRESS DOWN.

COLOR THIS ENTIRE PAGE.

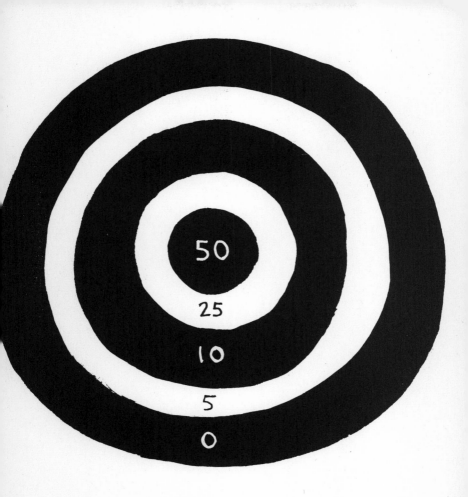

50
25
10
5
0

THROW SOMETHING
A PENCIL, A BALL DIPPED IN PAINT.

# SCRATCH

USING A SHARP OBJECT.

# DO SOME RUBBINGS WITH A PENCIL.

# SCRIBBLE WILDLY, VIOLENTLY, with RECKLESS ABANDON.

# TEAR STRIPS
## RIP IT UP!

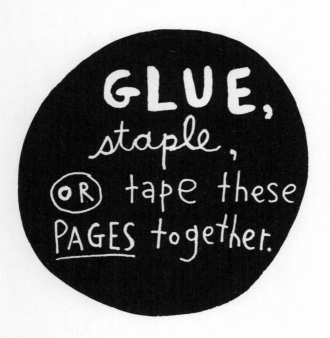

*draw lines*

ON THE BUS, ON

While IN MOTION,
RAIN, WHILE WALKING.

# FILL THIS PAGE WITH CIRCLES.

Document your dinner.

RUB, SMEAR, SPLATTER YOUR FOOD.

USE THIS PAGE AS A NAPKIN.

# CHEW ON this.

↓

*WARNING: DO NOT SWALLOW.

# MAKE A FUNNEL.

DRINK SOME WATER.

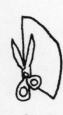
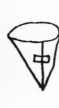
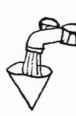

1. CUT OUT.

2. ROLL & TAPE.

3. ADD WATER & DRINK.

TEAR OUT

# CRUMPLE.

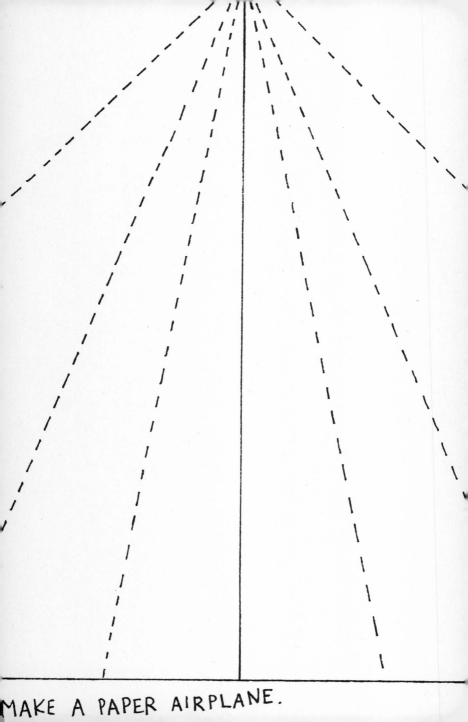

MAKE A PAPER AIRPLANE.

like
this

# WRAP something

## WITH THIS PAGE.

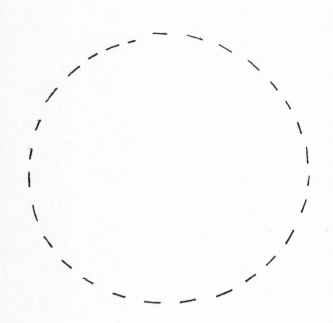

# TONGUE PAINTING

1. EAT SOME COLORFUL CANDY.

2. LICK THIS PAGE.

WRITE ONE WORD

OVER AND OVER.

**TIE** A STRING TO THE *spine* OF THIS BOOK.

# SWING WILDLY

LET IT HIT THE WALLS.

PICK UP THE JOURNAL WITHOUT USING YOUR HANDS.

CLIMB
UP HIGH
DROP THE
JOURNAL.

compost this page.

watch it deteriorate

# DO A really UGLY
(USE UGLY SUBJECT MATTER
A BADLY DRAWN BIRD,

# DRAWING

(GUM, POO, DEAD THINGS, MOLD, BARF, CRUD.)

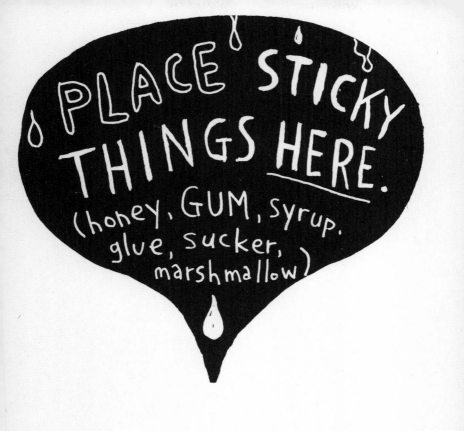

PRETEND YOU
ARE DOODLING
ON THE BACK
OF AN ENVEL-
OPE WHILE
ON THE PHONE.

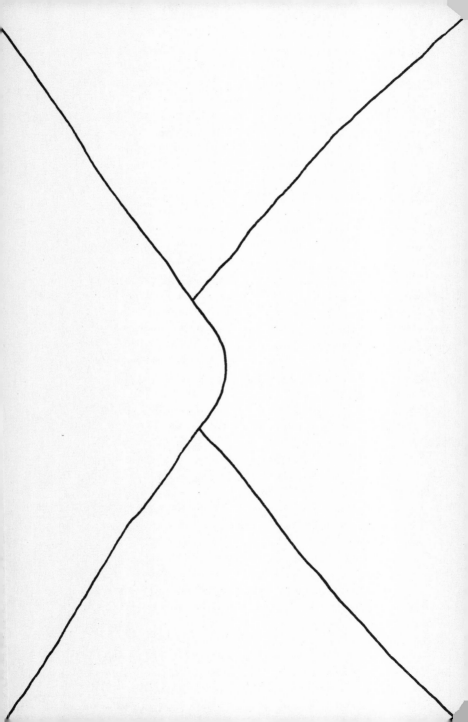

# JOURNAL GOLF

1. TEAR OUT PAGE. CRUMPLE INTO A BALL.
2. PLACE JOURNAL INTO A TRIANGLE SHAPE.
3. HIT/KICK THE BALL THROUGH THE TRIANGLE.

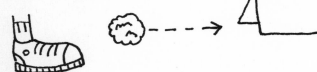

make a paper chain.

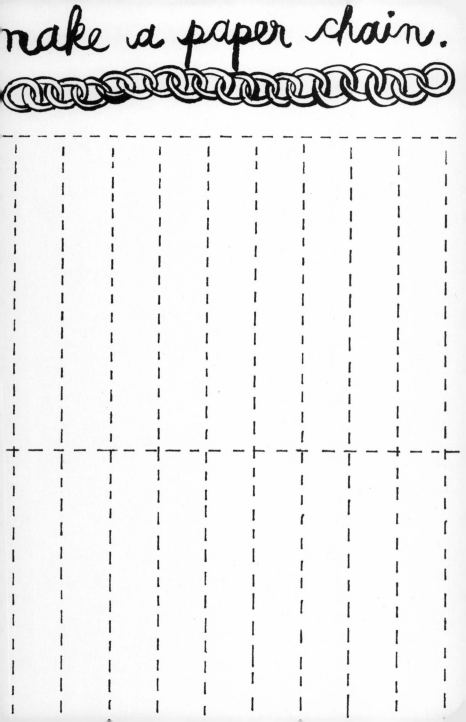

COLLECT
FRUIT
STICKERS*
HERE.

*STICKERS YOU FIND ON BOUGHT FRUIT.

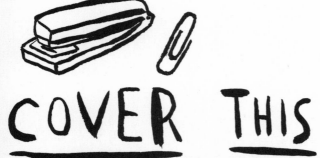

COVER THIS PAGE

JSING ONLY OFFICE SUPPLIES.

# BRING THIS BOOK IN THE SHOWER WITH YOU.

GO FOR A WALK, DRAG IT.

TIE A STRING TO THE JOURNAL.

RUB HERE WITH DIRT.

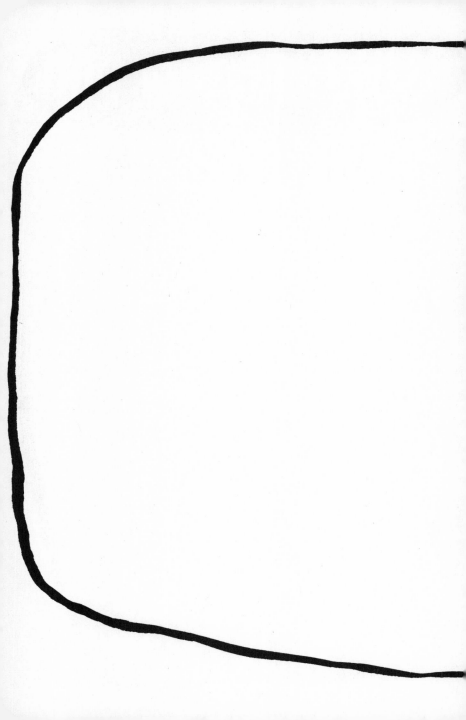

USE THIS AS A

*test Page*

FOR PENS, PAINTS,
MARKERS, OR ART SUPPLIES.

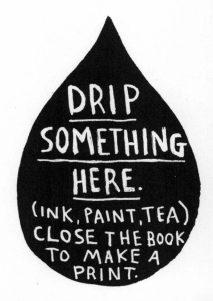

DRIP
SOMETHING
HERE.
(INK, PAINT, TEA)
CLOSE THE BOOK
TO MAKE A
PRINT.

Sew this page

glue A RANDOM PAGE FROM A NEWSPAPER HERE.

A PLACE FOR YOUR GROCERY LISTS.

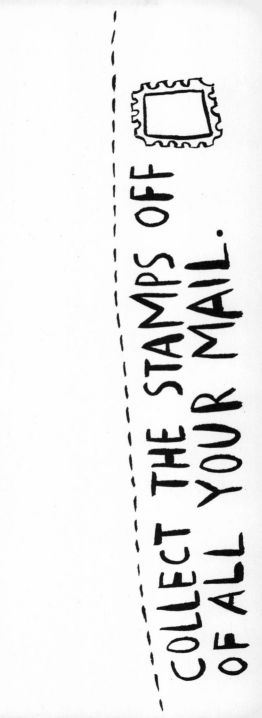

COLLECT THE STAMPS OFF OF ALL YOUR MAIL.

TRACE THE THINGS
IN YOUR BAG (OR POCKETS).
LET THE LINES OVERLAP.

COVER THIS PAGE

WITH WHITE THINGS.

scribble wildly using only borrowed pens.

(document where they were borrowed from.)

MAKE A SUDDEN, DESTRUCTIVE, UNPREDICTABLE MOVEMENT WITH THE JOURNAL.

MAKE A MESS,
CLEAN IT UP.

DOODLE OVER TOP OF:

- ☐ THE COVER.
- ☐ THE TITLE PAGE.
- ☐ THE INSTRUCTIONS.
- ☐ THE COPYRIGHT PAGE.

FOLD DOWN THE CORNERS
OF YOUR FAVORITE PAGES.

Page of good thoughts.

MAKE PRINTS USING AN INK PA AND CUT VEGETABLES.

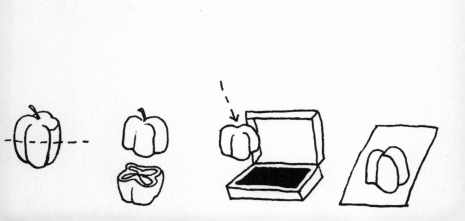

ASK A FRIEND TO DO SOMETHING DESTRUCTIVE TO THIS PAGE. DON'T LOOK.

# WRITE CARELESSLY. NOW.

Carelessly...

# GLUE RANDOM ITEMS HERE.
(i.e., things you find in your couch, on the street, etc.)

# tear this page out.

PUT IT IN YOUR POCKET.
PUT IT THROUGH THE WASH.
STICK IT BACK IN.

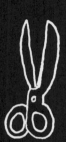

CUT
THROUGH
SEVERAL
LAYERS

Infuse this page with a smell of your choosing.

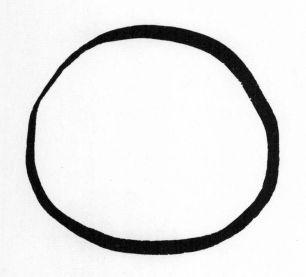

COLOR OUTSIDE
OF THE LINES.

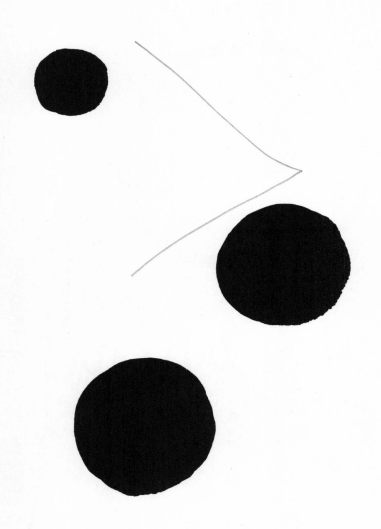

CLOSE YOUR EYES.

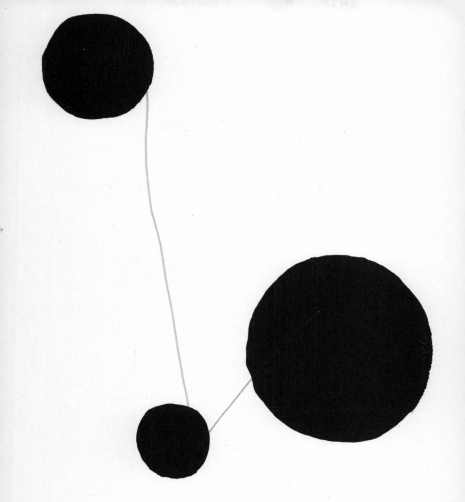

CONNECT THE DOTS
FROM MEMORY.

HANG THE JOURNAL IN A PUBLIC PLACE.
INVITE PEOPLE TO DRAW HERE.

# COLLECT YOUR

GLUE IT HERE

↓ ↓ ↓ ↘

# POCKET LINT.

trace **YOUR** hand.

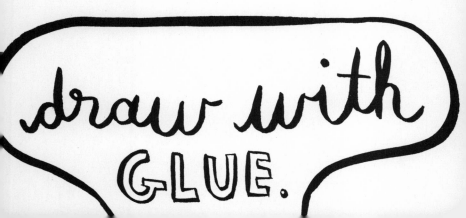

draw with GLUE.

# SAMPLE VARIOUS SUBSTANCES FOUND IN YOUR HOME.

DOCUMENT WHAT THEY ARE.
CREATE COLOR THEMES.

# DOCUMENT A BORING

# EVENT IN DETAIL.

CREATE A DRAWING USING A PIECE (OR SEVERAL PIECES) OF YOUR HAIR.

STICK PHOTO
HERE.

glue in a photo of
yourself you dislike.
DEFACE.

# DRAW <u>LINES</u> USING
WRITING UTENSILS
(STICKS, SPOONS, TWIST TIE

ABNORMAL

IPPED IN INK OR PAINT.

OMB, ETC.)

fill in this page when you are really ANGRY.

# WRITE OR DRAW

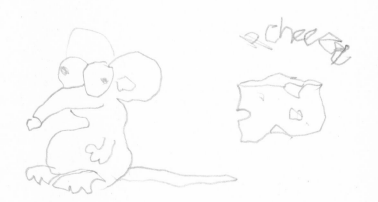

cheese

WITH YOUR LEFT HAND.

FIND A
WAY TO
WEAR THE
JOURNAL.

this page is a sign.
what do you want it to say?

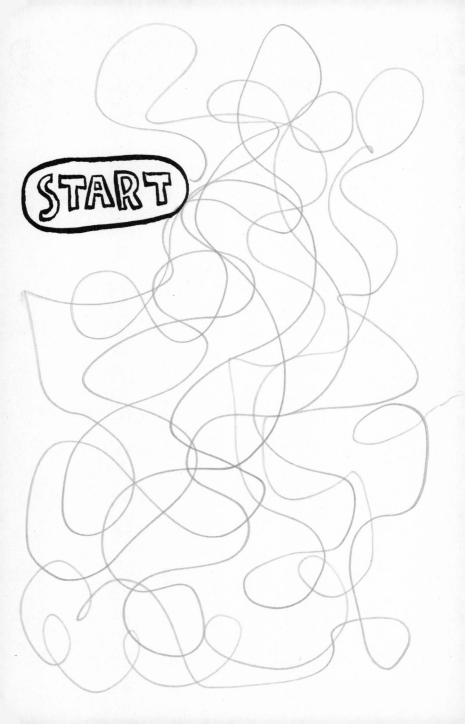

CREATE A NONSTOP
LINE.

# SPACE FOR NEGATIVE COMMENTS.*

* WHAT IS YOUR INNER CRITIC SAYING?)

DRAW LINES
WITH YOUR
PEN OR
PENCIL.
LICK YOUR FINGER
AND SMEAR
THE LINES.

# LOSE THIS PAGE.

(THROW IT OUT.)

ACCEPT THE LOSS.

# A PAGE for FOUR-LETTER WORDS.

GLUE IN A PAGE FROM A MAGAZINE.

CIRCLE WORDS YOU LIKE.

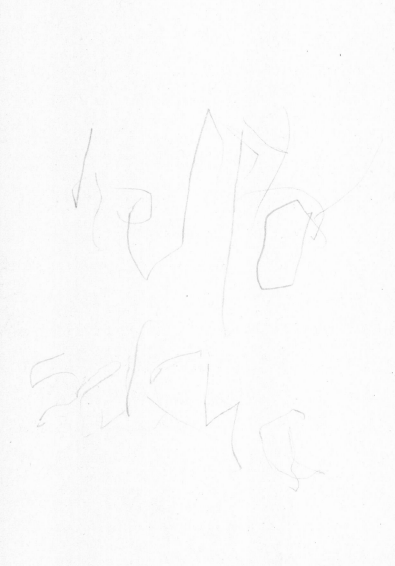

write with the pen in your mouth.

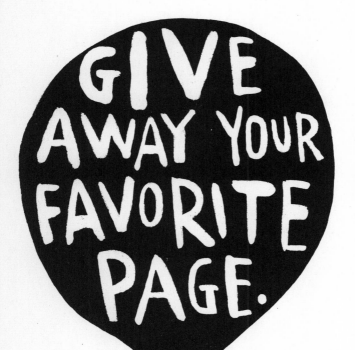

GIVE AWAY YOUR FAVORITE PAGE.

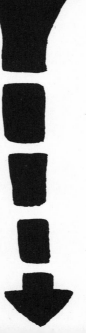

.drawkcab etirW

THIS SPACE IS DEDICATED

TO INTERNAL MONOLOGUE.

SCRUB THIS PAGE.

HIDE A SECRET MESSAGE SOMEWHERE IN THIS BOOK.

SLEEP WITH THE JOURNAL

Describe the experience here.)

CLOSE THE JOURNAL.

WRITE/SCRIBBLE SOMETHING ON THE EDGES.

WRITE A LIST OF MORE WAYS TO
WRECK THIS JOURNAL.

1.

2.

3.

4.

5.

6.

7.

8.

9.

10.

11.

12.

# STAIN LOG

# DOODLE OVER TOP OF THIS PAGE ↓↓↓ AND IN THE MARGINS.

This is not an important piece of writing. The author of this work is writing with the intention of creating a body of text that has little or no meaning. It is merely a texture of sorts that the reader will view as a canvas. Hopefully it will simulate a book that is embedded in your memory, a book you had in your childhood, the one that you secretly wrote in with your crayons. Maybe you were scolded for this by someone.

It could be your first textbook, which you defaced with your pen, prompted by the previous owner's little scrawlings. It was not your fault. Textbooks are destined to be defaced, it is a part of their nature. You are not to be blamed. Anything as boring as a textbook deserves everything it gets.

Are you reading this? You are supposed to be defacing this page. Please stop reading at once! This is your chance to deface something.

Maybe it is not as alluring because you are being told to do it. In that case I command you to cease your drawing immediately! If you make one more mark on this page the author will personally ban you from reading any future books of hers, in perpetuity (or for as long as she continues to make books, which will probably be for a very long time).

There are many things that you could do in place of defacing this page that would be more benefi-cial. Some examples include going to the dentist, cleaning out your fridge, washing the windows, cleaning under your bed, reading the entire works of Proust, arranging your food alphabetically, conducting a scientific study of polymer synthesis and its effects on the world, arranging your envelopes according to size, counting how many sheets of paper you have in your possession, making sure that all of your socks have partners, documenting your pocket lint (oh, yes you already did that earlier in this book), calling your mother back, learning to speak a new language, recording yourself sleeping, moving your furniture around to simulate a bus station, experimenting with new methods of sitting that you've never tried before, jogging on the spot for an hour, pretending you are a secret agent, decorating the inside of your fridge, drawing a fake door on your wall with chalk, conversing with your animal neighbors, writing a speech for a future award, walking to the corner store as slowly as possible, writing a positive feedback letter to your mail delivery person, putting a secret note into a library book, practicing finger strengthening exercises, dressing up as your favorite author, smelling the inside of your nose, memorizing *The Elements of Style* by Strunk and White, sitting on your front porch with a sign that says "Honk if you love birds," documenting the plants in your life on paper, smelling this book, sleeping, pretending to be a famous astronaut.

FIGURE OUT A WAY TO ATT ACH THESE TWO PAGES TOGETHER.

RUB THIS PAGE ON A DIRTY CAR.

COLLECT
THE LETTER
"W"
HERE.

**X** COLLECT
DEAD
BUGS
HERE.

DRUM ON THIS
PAGE WITH PENCILS.

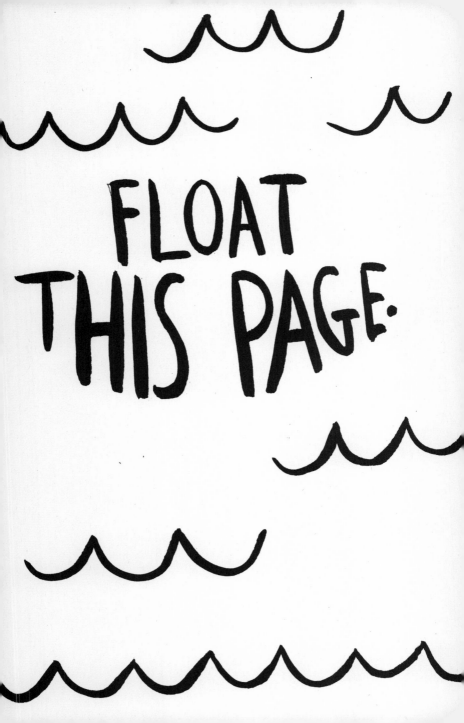

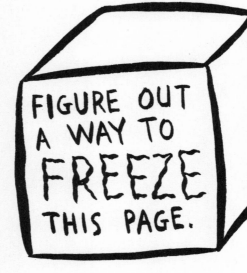

# HIDE THIS PAGE IN YOUR NEIGHBOR'S YARD.

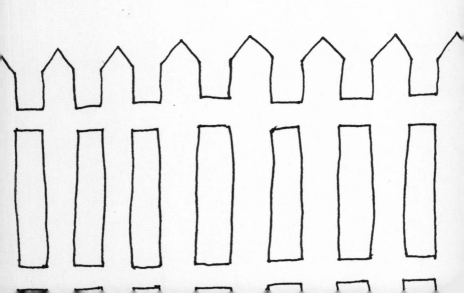

ROLL THE JOURNAL DOWN A LARGE HILL.

SELL
THIS
PAGE.

SLIDE THE JOURNAL
(THIS PAGE FACE-DOWN),
DOWN A LONG HALLWAY.

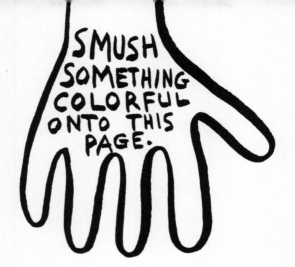

SMUSH
SOMETHING
COLORFUL
ONTO THIS
PAGE.

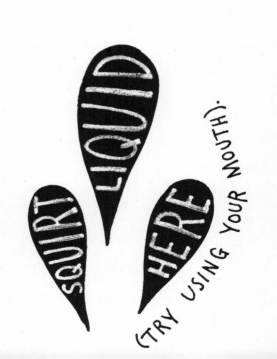
SQUIRT LIQUID HERE (TRY USING YOUR MOUTH).

COVER THIS PAGE IN TAPE

(CREATE SOME KIND OF PATTERN).

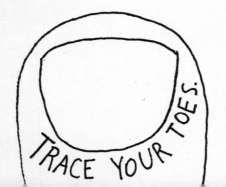

TRACE YOUR TOES.

# ALSO FROM KERI SMITH

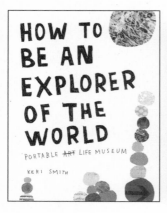

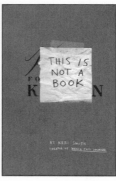

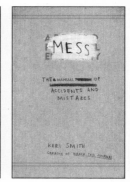

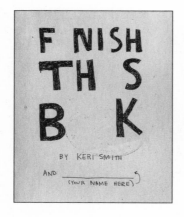

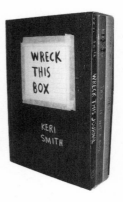

FOR MORE INFORMATION, VISIT
PENGUIN.COM/KERISMITH • PENGUIN.COM/WRECKTHISAPP